SOMATIC

Also by Ann Keniston

Poetry

November Wasps (chapbook)

The Caution of Human Gestures

Prose

Ghostly Figures: Memory and Belatedness in Postwar American Poetry

Overheard Voices: Address and Subjectivity in Postmodern American Poetry

Edited Volumes

Ethics after Poststructuralism: A Critical Reader
(with Brendan Johnston and Lee Olsen)

The News from Poems: Essays on 21ˢᵗ-Century American Poetry of Engagement(with Jeffrey Gray)

*The New American Poetry of Engagement:
A 21ˢᵗ-Century Anthology* (with Jeffrey Gray)

Literature after 9/11 (with Jeanne Follansbee Quinn)

SOMATIC

Ann Keniston

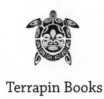

Terrapin Books

Terrapin Books
4 Midvale Avenue
West Caldwell, NJ 07006

www.terrapinbooks.com

ISBN: 978-1-947896-25-3
LCCN: 2020930165

First Edition

Cover art by Suzanne Sbarge
Sky Port
mixed media on panel

www.suzannesbarge.com

In memory of my mother

CONTENTS

somatic: of, relating to, or affecting the body

psychosomatic: of, relating to, concerned with, or involving both mind and body or relating to, involving, or concerned with bodily symptoms caused by mental or emotional disturbance

—Merriam-Webster Dictionary

A Note on Somatic Illnesses

This collection explores the discourse surrounding so-called psychosomatic illnesses, that is, illnesses that manifest through somatic or bodily symptoms. It is sometimes difficult to distinguish the psychosomatic from the physiological (or purely somatic), an ambiguity often framed in moral terms, since the psychosomatic is considered less real than the physiological. Hysteria, now called conversion disorder, makes this tension especially evident.

The poems in this volume, especially in the second and third sections, are informed by debates and discussions about hysteria over the past century and a half and especially by writings about Anna O., the famous Viennese "first hysteric" treated by Josef Breuer between 1880 and 1882. Anna was the daughter of a rigid, piously Jewish father who died just after Anna's symptoms emerged. These symptoms, which included partial paralysis, "absences," deafness, and aphasia, prevented her from attending to him. Breuer notes but does not elaborate on this fact, the Oedipus complex not yet having been invented, though he did devise a treatment Anna named "the talking cure," involving daily visits, during which Breuer encouraged Anna to tell elaborate "sad," and "very pretty" tales.

Breuer's writeup of his treatment of Anna was published as the first case study in *Studies on Hysteria* (1895), a volume Breuer cowrote with his then-protégé Sigmund Freud. Anna's case became central to Freud's still-developing theories of repression, infantile sexuality, and transference. Yet the published case history wasn't an accurate account of Anna's illness and treatment, as H. F. Ellenberger demonstrated in 1972: Breuer had earlier written a longer, and till then unpublished, version of the case history, which acknowledged the treatment's failure, partly due to Breuer's overprescription of morphine and chloral, to which Anna was addicted when the treatment abruptly ended.

Ellenberger also learned that Anna was the pseudonym of Bertha Pappenheim, an eminent feminist and social worker concerned with improving the lives of unmarried women and their children, so renowned that her image posthumously adorned a 1954 German postage stamp. Bertha was also an accomplished lacemaker and a poet and writer of children's stories that recall the fanciful tales Breuer encouraged her to invent during their treatment. As an adult, Bertha apparently never acknowledged her hysteria or treatment but always expressed strong contempt for psychoanalysis.

In the decades since Ellenberger's discoveries, Anna's story has been reinterpreted in a wide range of creative and scholarly ways. Her illness has been variously attributed to malingering (pretending to be ill); a "folie à deux," in which she developed symptoms to satisfy her over-eager doctor, who in turn demanded more elaborate symptoms; medical conditions from epilepsy to tubercular meningitis to schizophrenia; overexposure to stage performances of mesmerism and other dubious magic show-like tricks common at the time; and, perhaps most often, Anna's repressive patriarchal family and culture.

Several poems in this collection also draw on the work of Jean-Martin Charcot, among the first doctors to treat hysterics (identified by him as "hystero-epilepsy"). Charcot's treatments at Paris's Salpêtrière Hospital included weekly public performances by the hysterical girls, some attended by Freud; Sarah Bernhardt and other celebrities were also often in attendance. Charcot reportedly rescued the hospital's hysterics from virtual seclusion, though some argue that his interest in their symptoms encouraged exaggeration; many images of the Salpêtrière hysterics remain, caught on camera, a new technology that some call essential to the development of hysteria.

Charcot argued that many so-called religious mystics were hysterical, but he acknowleged, toward the end of his life that trips to Lourdes, famous for its miraculous curative powers, might help otherwise incurable hysterics. Many of the hysterics in his care, the definitive volume describing them indicates, were orphans who were sexually abused as children.

Somatic is also informed by my interest in the forms of ode and elegy; I am especially concerned with the blurring and overlapping of these traditionally opposed modes. The aria, a form I borrow from opera, strikes me as an especially hysterical form, and I use it to speak in the voice of an Anna-like hysteric in the third section of the collection.

This collection is indebted to the scholars who have discussed Anna's case and hysteria more generally; several of these poems are in dialogue with their writings, from which I sometimes cite in italics. Because hysteria often manifests itself through a dysregulation of speech and logic, several poems take liberties with syntax in ways consistent with Anna's speech as transcribed by Breuer, some of which I also cite in the "Verbatim" section of "Aphasic." In fact, preexisting symptoms, images, and texts are often recombined in hysteria, and while the successful treatment of hysteria (and modern-day conversion disorder) involves untangling them, that process sometimes leads to even more entanglement.

LAMENT / PRAISE: ELEGIES

The ode just visible beneath the elegy
The preemptive elegy
                    —Ben Lerner

Opaque

And then my mother wasn't

there. Not translucent, then
transparent, like the girl's hand
in the movie. Nor was she diffused

or reabsorbed by me

or stored in condensed form
for later or a pure idea
just past where I could see.

I couldn't cram her

into me, not a single
fleck, splinter or sweet
or painful memory that used to

make me cry, nor fill the holes

I'd made her make
in me. There was no creaking
deus ex machina or

electronic gizmo to bring

her back, though her absence
was a thing, immaterial
because gone, an idea

of the concept of the absence

of what was never solid
or still, like looking
into a camera obscura,

which reproduces everything

upside down, backward
and inconstantly, the image made
of light, unreproducible

unless someone chooses

a single moment
to preserve and undertakes
the labor of transcribing it.

UNCONSCIOUS

In each of us, my mother thought,
there exists a hidden essence, mostly evident

as pain or desire or the compulsion to repeat,
not immortal soul but the unconscious. Now that, as

others say, she's passed, I like to visit churches
that display the uncorrupted remains of saints

and their sculpted bodies, the garment hems
smooth from being touched. No one but Bernadette

could see the beautiful smiling child in white
who called herself Immaculate, but thousands

came to Lourdes to watch her witnessing
that miracle. The blind, lame, and dying still

arrive in buses. Past the kitschy shops, the spring
Bernadette scrabbled in the dirt to find,

and the porch cluttered with abandoned
canes and wheelchairs, they press their hair

and faces against the muddy wall,
the enormous church behind them

affirming an uncontaminated world
in the midst of escalating misery and also

the body in pain. I don't believe my mother
is immortal or scattered over the earth

or even alive in me. But in dreams, which let
the unconscious speak in puns and symbols,

she sometimes returns, often thin and naked
but occasionally healthy, wearing

her elegant work clothes. Sometimes she sits with me
beside a hanging garden whose flowers,

because they are so heavy, bloom abundantly,
their weight enabling the blooming, then

greater heaviness and more blooming.

ANTIDOTE

Let lack
be everything.

Inside, there's
nothing

but transparency,
not means

nor end nor
shape. Let

emptiness rise up
in her and fill

what never could
be filled.

She liked to save
new clothes because

to wait brings
pleasure, small

jangle of the hangers,
all the tags

still on
till it was time. Now

we have no time,
which means we have

forever, so let's wait
a little longer

till the soup's
grown cold and we're

no longer hungry.
Soon she'll start

to touch my injuries,
not to defend herself

or hurt me
but as an antidote

to harm. O
I am burning

sick. I cannot
eat or drink

or speak so let me
cling this little

while. How
dry and cool

her hands are
on my brow.

And now she lays
an icy cloth

here where
I'm on fire

and lets me
climb into her bed

and stay there
all night long.

TETHERED

*The open secret registers the subject's accommodation
to a totalizing system that has obliterated the difference
he would make.*
                    —D. A. Miller

My first accommodation
was pretending not to see
the thing I knew my mother

was most ashamed of.
As if my silence
could protect her, be

a wall or frame or
homely, homemade
structure we could live

inside forever. Sometimes
the dirt and leaves came in.
Sometimes we joked about

how cold we got and
held each other tight
though I didn't like

to touch. I thought to name
her secret or split it open
would hurt her

more. But even if I'd
yelled or wept or recognized
the secret was an almost

harmless set of actions
she inflicted mostly on
herself, it probably

would have made
no difference. Nor
could I ever have unmade

the totalizing system
she thought she had invented,
then adapted to

her own requirements, then
obliterated the way out.
She hid almost all

the traces of that thing
till it existed only
in the diagnostic

or judgmental language we
disliked, her silence a way
she tried to shield me

from what was worse
except I eavesdropped
and sneaked looks.

Now nothing's left
but a mass of what
were once her cells

or less than that.
My loyalty's set around
sheer space, her story

just another
of a woman's body
unable to resist.

But still, too late,
I hide the details, as if
her secret had a form

as she once did or were
a tether joining us, a way
I still can hold her close.

Injured

Having been cut
so many times

her flesh grew numb

so she created
a pretend baby
she couldn't love
without crushing

and failed to bring it
to breast because she
was starving—

as when God
forced his son
to sacrifice his son

then sacrificed his own

having suffered
all the children
to come unto him

suffering

the mortal
envelope

curtain she sewed
with her body
and hid behind

then again cut her fingers
with her hands

AMENDS

If I could make amends, repair
the harm I've done, received,
be free from faults,

I would beg on my knees,
pull off the itchy shirt, forswear
the tin cup, lies
and greed

and disavow my flaws,
stain or blemish—

or stand beside the marsh
in late light

having been repaid, cured,
the antidote already in my hands

which are empty, having
abandoned

all the hoarded goods,
the folded paper
corrected and made accurate,

illegible with damp.

NEST

Italicized words borrowed from writings
by Henry James, Sr.

A nest   of mud and straw
shaped by the body   of the bird
raveled   and raveling
there   where it came to rest
even a *vastation*   has a body
squatting   in a corner
a refuge   in unenclosed space
in that game where we fell   into each other's arms
released we thought   by air
so wounded   that man said
he couldn't hire   or cure or care
nor grant me anymore her   *No*
but now permit   occasionally
an egret   to appear
among the ducks   and geese
and for a while   exist
on earth   S-shaped
in muck   probing for
what's lost   o unhook
the remainder   from the light
let leaves fall down   onto my shoulders
over weeks   having yellowed
gotten loose

UNLOVABLE

There was a year or several when I thought my mother
was punishing me for a flaw I couldn't see

or way I'd hurt her. All the years since then,
that error reproduced itself, changed form

and object. And then I saw she'd done her best
but was so hurt. After my friend's divorce,

her daughter grew so anxious she could hardly
speak. The change, she called it. The transition.

She quit her new job and in the afternoons
they sat together on the sofa or sometimes

went to the movies. I thought I was unlovable,
then unloved, which was also wrong.

In the silent movie, my parents walk in
laughing, my mother's hand on my father's shoulder,

both of them so casually tender just a few years
before he left her. Often, the neutral scene

is streaked with flame. But there must also exist
a place that isn't harmed. Like the salmon

arrowing upstream through the roil
of water pushing them back down—

from the special viewing window,
it seemed they hardly moved.

ASH

Italicized words borrowed from
Anne Carson's *Economy of the Unlost*

The chord
the train horn makes

is shorn
of touch. As for

the poplars beside
Monet's Seine,

light interferes,
not overlay or depth

but another surface
to try to paint.

Always the emblem
of vanishing repeats.

It was made
to be released. Ash

trickles out
through fingers

till there remains
no burnished edge

or residue of silt,
splayed limbs or

earth's embrace.
One's hands unclench

their grip. I had
an original but left it out

too long in rain
so made this replica with what

was left: unloved
nest, moth, some leaves

above the lake that makes
a mirror

I require
and cannot bear,

still standing
inside hunger, abandoned

there, already there when
the flame burned down.

Redundant

I must have loved her weakness

when she began to weaken

when everyone was harmed

the humiliations exposed themselves

some daily and mundane humiliations

too expensive to contain

inside I found a seed

like seeds embedded in a raspberry

like a bird with a broken wing

as if what were valuable had been broken

as if what is costly has been repaired

the cost is holding secrets in

as if the parts could be glued

the glued-together parts exist

so I can make an elegy

so I can write an ode

an ode entwined around unloveliness

an elegy untethered

detached from its object.

ELEGY ODE

Italicized words borrowed from various
definitions of the ode

To string together extant
words or phrases
                    in
irregular form

                        makes
this awkward

thing, half song half
garment with
                seams

exposed
            then *rent,*

                        unless
a facsimile is built
from shards, then
invoked:

            O muse
or doctor,
unnamed absent one,

you secret self:
                please sit
with me a little longer beside

the darkness
underlying all.

DISPLACEMENT: ODES

The hysteric's body is a site for displacement; hysteria, like photography, produces a snippet of "truth" in the form of a symptom.
                    —Mady Schutzman

DISPLACED

Into each space I stuck
a word, then something else

like a cup left out in rain. Often
they were misconstrued, my

offhand remarks or lies. So I took
a day job: first I learned to yield, then

held up the YIELD sign.
What mattered was the repeated

gesture of brushing off or
shooing, what is sometimes called

displacement. I knew the ode was drifting
past where I could rescue it,

and I pitied everything I couldn't
hold inside it, all the abandoned things

and phrases, shirt, glue gob, tiny spider.
That's why I let some stranger

pull my lips apart, pour in
some sounds and stroke me

till I swallowed. I mean I'm not
the one who made me rehearse.

Who bade, then made me sing.

SOMATIC

So I could let her in
                    and spill

my secret animosity and

sweet, I found some other
broken girls I hadn't known
existed till she
                    got lost to me, lacy

wraiths I pitied first, then came
to love since all they had

were bodies and the body's
requirements come both first
and last. Illness is another

form of speech,
                    somatic, enmeshed
in flesh and manifest as symptom
and release,

                    a code
I also speak, their voices
my portion, penance, snippet,

violent or tender but
                    always loyal

since all I wanted
was not to further harm

my fragile, lost, familiar one.

CONCORDANCE

Salpêtrière Hospital, Paris, 1880

On Tuesday afternoons, the bodies of mute
    or paralyzed hysterics twitched, then moaned

on cue before a crowd, then all alone made love
    while mesmerized. A touch or pressure *there*

could make asymptomatic girls convulse, then
    deliver each from all her symptoms.

In photographs, a graceful girl in white raises
    an arm while falling. Her chemise is loose.

The doctors clustered round, hysteria the sheet
    they used to shroud, then touch that trembling.

No protocol or rubric existed yet to translate
    what they saw despite their patient searching

for a key or at least a concordance to what
    they must have known they'd never fully master,

just some words to put beside those gestures, each
    almost-theory disproven by the newest batch

of symptoms till psychoanalysis became a curtain
    filled with holes and also light. Or else the truth

existed somewhere else. Uncured, most girls
    remained locked in. A few got work in traveling shows

acting out their formerly uncontrollable symptoms
    before an audience that paid. Crowds still line up

to watch the newest pretty girl impelled
    to go to sleep, then rise up from bed, rigid,

cataleptic, like the blurry girls in those old photos,
       her hands askew and stuck. And then the man—

call him magician or doctor of throwing out
       into the dark—waves his hands to prove there is

no transparent shelf or set of ropes, then covers
       then makes her disappear till she emerges

from the wings unharmed, which means it's time
       for everyone to applaud at that old trick

made new, then surge into the aisles
       and go back home to dreams that if

remembered gesture toward the same
       old mystery. In mine last night I stood

inside a ring of brambles hidden in wild grass.
       And then a staircase spiraled up, unanchored,

like the stairs in fairy tales or myths.

CONVERSION

And then I made
an actual girl, hysterical,

from husks
and scattered pages

and her dust.
I licked her lips

and then her scar,
hurt bruise,

bereaved, her
hiding place. I mean

she was a house
I squatted in

and found some random
stuff to bind

with string and told
to dance and

danced with her
till she became my voice,

reed, oboe, syrinx, flute,
her loose

unmothered mutterings
in my mouth,

scant, then
scattered over the fields,

leaving me free
to stare into

the windless
pond of her, redoubled

pale and faltering
in her glass.

INSCRIBED

Morgellons Disease

According to its laws

the afflicted body speaks in different
tongues

until eventually
one's fingers find

some bits inscribed
in the delicate skin
of the inner arm or belly

and scrape them out

the body incomplete till
marred by one's own hand

which is how mourning
goes underground, displaced

or else it's *mass hysteria,* a delusion
transmitted by Internet

though the experts

like the skeptical compelled to touch
Jesus' wounds
and then St Francis'

can't stop marveling at
the fantastical symptoms.

PROPHYLACTIC

Munchausen Syndrome by Proxy

A bruise on
the scalp

or burn or injection
                    it was said
loosens the knot

for whoever comes next, just
another mother inventing
the same solution

to impose on her most
beloved child because

she lacks other tools—

*

a prophylactic injury,
preventing something worse

or a cure
ahead of time, like bestowing
on one's body just

a little cut to excise
the impulse to obliterate it altogether—

*

which leaves an excess
of evidence,
                    so many photos

the judge and jury
used to construct an argument
                          in favor

of a diagnosis otherwise unproved

*

till the diagnosis, like
an actual object under
pressure
          buckles

and must be removed
from the medical manuals

since when desire's involved

who knows
what's real, those erstwhile

perpetrators only ever
victims eventually

released from prison, blinking
in the bleached
light, as newspaper photographs
                          confirm.

SIMULATION

Italicized words borrowed from discussions of
Anna's case by Breuer and Michel Borch-Jacobson

and then: a contracture
of the wrists and ankles

not less real
for being simulated

because it is necessary to be consumed
by *the whole business*

and then report *she had not been ill*
at all

*

she watches the mechanical
angel

a simulated girl

because
that is her part: to watch
its inability

to move its wings

*

an ordinary girl can't move her wings
unless someone arrives,
                              deus

ex machina, and opens them

with levers and gears, the way
it once was done, a re-

enactment by machine, a happy
accident, gentle

handed as she might
have been.

ECHO

Italicized words borrowed from Breuer's case
history of Anna O.

when the patient is *merely*
the doctor's *echo*

that commonplace mimeticism

assuming their respective roles:
the symptoms

returning *again and again*

to the problem of
what we call 'suggestion'

a double or doubling
overlapping

suggestion
may have contaminated the whole

or his *own echo*

because she was *already*
hysterical, entranced
and unstable

in certain performances

and that goes double
for Breuer

in retrospect: a book

small or handmade

to be brought into bed and opened

like bolts of cloth spread in a shop

and for each thing, two words

the second beginning *un*

roughly translated: love, his
own echo pressed onto the illness

a stamp or mark, impure
because there was no alternative:

please take
this *unstable* offering

Symptomatic: Anna's Arias

Hysteria gives us the maximal conversion of psychic affect into somatic meaning—meaning enacted on the body itself. . . . The aria offers us at once the hysterical impasse and the working through of that impasse.
—Peter Brooks

OPERATIC

Italicized words borrowed from Peter Brooks's
"Body and Voice in Melodrama"

Often, there arrives a break in the action
for even the most stubborn girl

                                        so an aria
can come, granting form
to *the hysterical impasse*

within the extant form
of *melodrama*

and filled with *distortions,
displacements, condensations, recounted dreams
and the rest*

                by which her *body*
makes *meaning* from
its leavings—

her stuttered or
half-swallowed borrowed words
mostly incomprehensible

each high note a coin
her secret palm
hides while pretending
to relinquish it

doubling and then again
the little she started with

till roses
cover the bare boards.

APHASIC

[Anna O.] lost her command of grammar and syntax;
she no longer conjugated verbs, and eventually used only
infinitives, for the most part incorrectly formed from
weak past participles . . . In the process of time, she
became almost completely deprived of words . . . language
failed her; she could find no tongue in which to speak.
                              —Josef Breuer

1. Verbatim

not totally deprived
to speak the other

languages, I learn anew

the but too well
motivated fear
to lose

2. Etiology

Who broke
              the frame

the pronouns not
in certain
              tongues:
no-thing
              nor
am understood, tongue

on the pillow I
embroidered when.

My *aphasic jargon* relieves
the need. One gesture
                            speaks

a thousand to the bitter
fact:
        such a
lucky me, to have

some later symptoms
to translate to
a future gaze.

3. Mute

As yet not *castrated* nor

resistant nor
malingerer

nor sing nor having cut

with blades or artificial
wings

but rearrange
some furniture as was then

before, a before-
thought so I can reminisce
my former
lustrousness

the hips and uterus
never bellied forth

such a little *self-
repudiating form:*

an *"object"*
going off in all directions

4. Talk

My master starts me
with *stock phrases* and
I carry on

discrepant and too far and
unstop my vocal trill

the clot in me
that whirs

and sputter out in languages and song
what happened when

all well and left and good

until there comes another
mute and stuttering

or time for exiting.

Diagnostic

Please preserve my other names
between some sheets
as yet
     unwritten on
and diagnose my sick

with just one word

             yes you
my erstwhile doctor

let the record show
I failed to interpose

            nor told
and failed to hear
another word but fell

nor ever called for help

such a little heap

of suffering
        I bequeath
to science what you find

while an unforeseen
clump of later girls
weeps in some later
basement room

          beset
by the same condition

addiction tuberculosis
or *simulation:*

here's
where I was marred
and marked

      and
sat up all night

my disregarded book
           askew

my hysterical
        hands unable
to tat the squares of lace
I afterward was known for.

ANNOUNCEMENT

To be inhabited, one must burn
one's edge. Or like the first
duped girl
          made from dirt

return in different
form. There are so many
lilies to arrange. So many

hours to practice swaying while

the interloper's words
unfurl in ornamental
scrolls

          and word and deed
conjoin in my
immaculate flesh

a blob called *babe*
in my tender crook while
the other girls
                    adopt
the same positions

conturbatio, humilatio, meritatio

and kneel in cloistered
gardens

          dreaming of some dreamy
savior, healer, cure-all
engendered from our
secret parts

           touching
our feet, unwrapping
useless strips of linen, all our

mortal bindings.

STIGMATA

Lourdes, 1898

Marked, I am
unholy, touched

with mystery or shame
the better to receive

divine disease, these
wounds

*

Not motherless but might as well be
flood me now
imbue   reverse   inflame
my blood

*

My doctor loves to count
and photograph whereas

the Christ's desire is to take
toss and heal me

tear me open
remove my beating heart

*

Please to Lourdes allow
a pilgrimage and heal my mind
along the way with
tools that brought
disorder   my humiliation
faith   my knife divine

my thread my body
where they tangle

*

*Under hypnosis the doctor impelled a welt to rise on her skin
and blister and bleed and persist long after she woke believing
she had burned herself because he told her that.*

*

faith is requisite
to topsy-turvy observation
based science to whose
decks the storm
tossed doctors cling

*

that the cure is
symptom is hysteria's
incommensurable
mystery

*

forgive my old-fashioned mind
body problem

nothing remains but
these punctured hands
gesturing in the skeptical air

PROJECTED

I had no other home except

this nest of bleached and broken
bones

       nor broken
bow, the violin
of me unable not to slip

in and out of recollected light

nor fillip, dab or
beach with scudding blocks of foam

such a tender
              hatchling self I made
by hand

       my hands the lens and visible
array, malformed, projected
on some wall or empty
sheet hung down

              thrown forward, stretching
forth, a pantomime

old-fashioned border
on which to perch, flat not

deep because of hiding
for so long, my clothes and limbs
                   too wide
to fit in any book

not girl but wing ratio
the wind gets stuck in then

moves through

my hands manipulated by
an outside thing or
man,

    a pillow, then a cup
for pretend water
that fails to slake

so many loyalty oaths
and reminiscences

cast out, the pattern caught
until it goes.

ESTRANGEMENT

I let my life contain whatever he poured in,
my instructor of handicap, doctor of broken dishes
and water in the lungs, and made a pitcher
and drank from it because he had withdrawn
from feeling and affection though I sat and watched
until I couldn't anymore, foreign to myself,
removed from my abode, having gone abroad
and drove all day and night and tried again
to swallow the enormous powdery tablet
of his absence until the sublime was manifest
at the crest of the hill, my affect
displaced among the leaves
and dirt, neglected, sublimated and symbolic
till bereavement was my name and wrapper,
punctured core, invented sacrament no one cared
to share though the loss grew unfamiliar
as the brightly colored currency
of some strange country, not without value but
having fallen out of circulation
and again I pretended to dab his lips, my hands
the water and the cloth, my lips so dry.

BELATED

Italicized words borrowed from
a poem by Bertha Pappenheim

My talisman was always
in my hands, seatbelt
after a wreck

or just a bit of cloth
or voice I sometimes
heard. A figurine

like those arrayed
on my doctor's shelves.
Amulet. A charm.

A copy of a lost
original, he said, which
left me free, my thirst

a kind of spool
of thread I wound up
all those years, though

the law of memory
isn't cling to but
erase, not gradually

but in violent
little jolts. Without
the aftermath

effect, there would
have been no dividend
or payout, no reason

to endure so long.
My secret stuck me
back to what I

yearned to be. Because
it was my afterlife, I went in
whole hog, let

some just-invented
gizmo expose my preexisting
flaws. I was a string

on which a broken bow
must play, a violin
that wove the light.

I mean delay lit up
my screen, revealed
soft tissues, all my bones.

ENVOY

I permit you to release me now. There is
no need to displace or substitute
your voice or answer back to

names I granted you before
of avatar or sick or slick
unbottomed home or bird or moth
or heap of ash or buttoned up
or other girl. I ghosted you, invoked,
embodied you and made you
speak. I taught you all my tricks
until you made me dream
you were alive, then recollect

your flickering all day. You let me pinch
your lips till I believed I was

a magic-show assistant,
ventriloquist and voice. Best friend

and confidant, mommy, sister I never had,
my poisoner and antidote, whipping girl, victim
and my subterfuge, a darkly mirrored me
and all my ghosts—you waited

in the wings till it was time, then let me
reassemble you from bits

of lies or actual memories. It's time to cut

me off, be quiet, stop. Or turn
into someone less harmed

and mean, less vague, more vehement,
not mute. Let me let you go.

ASSEMBLAGE: ODES

Pattern born amid formlessness. . .
—James Gleick

ASSEMBLAGE

Today's lesson is: injury takes many
forms. And: healing is an act of will. Or artifice

or wall. A poem conceals its author's secrets
by giving them another form. Some artists

like to cut, then rearrange and glue
objects they pick up into new shapes. Or else

collect a bunch of scattered scraps they can't
align. Some women whose brains were cut

or suctioned felt grateful to be released
from the hospital's back wards though the doctor

made mistakes. In psychodrama workshops,
each grown-up child in turn must confront

the volunteer who plays her father,
telling him how it felt till the dad

confesses, repents, apologizes though he never did
in life. And then the participants join hands

to celebrate having lifted up their life-
long hurt together and let it go like

an actual fragile, bulky object
they hadn't known could float. Grief's

a necessary stage. If handled carefully, it can
heal. Or be sealed up. On television I watched

a female dancer clamber up into
her partner's arms and be let fall, then climb

back up and be let go again. Her falling
made a clattering. Eventually I realized

that series of gestures was a routine those dancers
had memorized. There was no actual harm.

Transmutation

The imagined Rapture in his novel
was, the author said, an allegory for 9/11

but focused not on grief or revenge,
since even after all those people disappeared

not much was different on Earth, the pessimists
still pessimistic, the repentants still wearing

special outfits while the bereft distracted themselves
with booze or sex. Maybe the law of conservation

of matter applies not just to disaster
but material things, and nothing's ever lost, just

changed in form, our loved ones in Heaven
still wearing the clothes they vanished in,

so distracted by whatever made them happiest
in life they hardly miss us. The actual planes, seen

by thousands, seemed to grow as they approached
the Towers, though that was an illusion.

The body keeps changing, not *transmutation*
or *transfiguration* but growth followed by

the breakdown of tissues and cells, the formerly
ripe parts drooping because it's time. Most

of the bodies of those killed on 9/11 were changed
into particles small enough to be inhaled, which

they were. In twenty or fifty years, probably no one
will recognize that novel's allusions,

artists long since having stopped trying to find
new ways to retell that story, a newer tragedy

by then having crowded out
the dimly recalled ones. We like to say

those who disappeared aren't really
gone as long as we remember them. There

remain so many emblems, not only
the fragile notices hung all over the city

those first days, some taken down and laminated
or projected onto the walls of the new museum

but all the possessions of the dead, some
also displayed, the ordinary jacket and gloves

important not because they are dust-covered
or burned or physically different in any way

but because they aren't, which is the point,
since our seeing changes them,

reveals they have been changed.

Multiple Version

1.

If God's a teacher, all
        His actions must
     instruct. When Isaac, the blameless

child, is brought up for sacrifice,
        the lesson is
     God's capricious. Or cruel or

in this case requires
        pure obedience
     in contradiction to

His juster law: *thou shalt*
        not kill. It's the kind
     of test abusers make

their victims take to prove
        their power
     is absolute. Does

He know His only son,
        the unborn one
     who'll save us all,

is marked for sacrifice?
        Maybe he stuck
     this plot twist in

to prove some mysteries
        can only be solved
     in retrospect.

2.

Mostly forgotten is the boy. Titian
          huddles him
    at the bottom of the frame,

almost in miniature, almost
           irrelevant, though
    he looks right at us while

the angel stays his father's
          hand. He's hard
    to notice amid

the upper fluttering
         of arms
    and wings. He knows

he is the sacrifice so
         loosened his own collar,
    pitying the perpetrator

as children do.

3.

Because I knew they had been
         hurt, I tried to serve
    my parents' weakness

through obedience. Now I see
         they were wrong
    to let me think love was a thing

I had to earn. I used to sit
         beside my father's bed
    while he slept, whole visits

I never told him about, free,
            I thought,
        from having to perform

obedience. But even unconscious,
            he defined
        the terms of my rebellion.

4.

My past transgressions
                diffuse. A butterfly
        effect: each one

becomes important somewhere
                else. Abraham was seen
        by God, the angel and

his son, so he existed
                in their sight.
        That mutual watching

opened us to ethics, which here
                means *mercy*.
        Sometimes I hold out a hand

to a friend or nearby stranger,
                not because I want
        to be a savior or even

nice but as if that almost
                inadvertent gesture
        could prevent me from

inflicting harm.

RESIDUE

Because it was too late to impose a moral
or chronicle the shards' provenance or rescue

some discarded thing from dust, I began
with what was left, the way great rectangular

Roman blocks were hauled off as *spolia*
and adapted to mundane purposes, a door jamb

or part of an arch or wall. To receive grace
doesn't mean believing you've been touched

by God. It's opening your arms to doubt,
the repeated non-appearance of

the longed-for proof until the faithful
gather on the porch to watch the lit-up hills

like a palette someone ought to lift
and paint with. Sometimes in stories all the pieces

come to life, the way the mute stones near
Orpheus' severed head wept to hear

its song, or the parts of Osiris' body, strewn
all over the world, clamored to be made whole

so again they could be scattered.

PROFUSION

Because my father could not walk, I dreamed
we walked beside a double lake where marsh birds

gathered in profusion, beautiful long-legged
waders visible without binoculars. And then

someone began to name them while the dusk
collapsed around us, but slowly, delaying

the dark, or I delayed it since I made
this scene, inserting light, then bits of dark

to fill the gaps. The girl who fell into an empty
pool and broke her spine didn't become

catatonic or brain-dead, not a cripple,
her mother thought, but a vessel made by God

for other people's suffering, a wick
or cipher, still and steadfast no matter

what she'd taken in. Most afternoons, the sick
gathered outside her window to watch her

on her special bed, thin-limbed, dressed
all in pink, until they felt, or thought

they felt, their pain lift away, then knelt
all over the lawn to worship her.

In my dream, my father thanked me but I knew
his pain continued, contained

and hidden by his bones and flesh like
something he refused to give me

out of mercy. Then we were driving
through the dark, the two of us exhausted,

until I found a stranger's house with people
sleeping everywhere, on beds and chairs, the floor.

Casually he walked in and lay down
and slept among them. This must be how I tally

what I haven't lost yet, lifting
each loved thing, then relinquishing it

to mourn its loss, redundantly desiring sleep
because I'm already sleeping. I had to wake

for the dream to do its work. And so I woke
and waited for the thin

November sunlight to enter the yard
while the leaves fell down in bunches and

two pairs of jays—deep blue,
oblivious—flashed between the trees.

FORMLESSNESS

Italicized phrases borrowed from
James Gleick's *Chaos: Making a New Science*

Formlessness came first, then dark, then light.

God gave us eyes to witness what he made

before he made us though *entropy* was already there,

a little cream swirling into *a cup of hot coffee*

a symptom of the forces of dispersal that preceded

form, though mostly we feel euphoric, not terrified

at *jagged edges* and *sudden leaps*. Formulas

explaining *coastlines*, extinctions, *traffic jams*

and *the arrhythmic writhing of a human heart in the moments*

before death contain so many *variables* they look

like random strings of letters and numbers but

are *beautiful* to those who understand

their fixed and open spaces where bits of order

lodge like mica flecks in granite or particles

that drift. Most astronomers *believe*, if not in God

then in the *deep structure* inside the *delicate structure*

of everything ever theorized or touched, and also

in *metaphor.* Even a casual observer of clouds

can detect *pattern amid formlessness* when damp air

rolls in over the high peaks, the clouds unregulated,

sometimes rising up in many-layered spirals, sometimes

in flat hollow discs, like smoke rings.

Sutured

As a torn paper might seal up its side,
Or a streak of water stitch itself to silk
—Howard Moss

1.

The sycamore has fastened itself
to light, inverted, tilting, its old bark
all over the grass. It flickers
in the afternoon. *Grief tree*, it has
been called. *The tree of sacrifice.*

*

There, where it broke, then healed, then broke again:
touch the suture, the imperfect
reassembly. Pull the staples out
and feel its former separateness.

*

A doctor knows where to find
the right material
because some cells can be draped
over the scaffold of muscle and bone
to regenerate in the dark.

*

Inside is some
ungrieving thing. Unhindered, known by heart,
which can't be touched
or plucked.

2.

inverted
grief tree:
pull out
the material
I can't pluck

*

I can't do without
where it broke:
suture, scaffold
fastened
to light

*

all over, grief: then
healed, then
imperfect reassembly

*

grief
I know by heart:
find some
ungrieving thing.

ULTIMATUM

Afterward, the heart
disobeys because something
has to break

and then be
reattached, fingers
pushing back

what tore because
we were once
one clay. Why not

unmake the law
that everything has to fall down
or decay, unmess

the messy room
using time-lapse
or play the film

backward so the flattened
man emerges
from under the steamroller

and walks away
unharmed? By now,
the barrier between us

is so thick
it's beautiful,
a lopsided, slippery,

topheavy, handmade
construction, threatening
to collapse, then

collapsing so we get
another chance to try
to repair it.

SYCAMORE

Permit me this
                redundancy. I dug
inside my bone to find
the right material, a fastener or dark.

Let me join me
                to myself
right here. And release
my unremarkable
heart.
          In myths, the fleeing girl
becomes a tree, the sacred tree,
the tree of patience. Again

the sycamore has spilled
its bark over the ground.

Here is where my invisible
begins. At the scar or border, lip,
my shore. My little wound has been
                                  sewn up
with thread.
                And look: the birds

are here, invisible but known.
Geese pass over in the night. Here

is where I was torn and then
remade. It is
both raw and smooth.

REASSEMBLY

To the intractable light

and tree limbs' shadows on the ceiling

and the gunk stuck onto things

I affixed my voice

*

I was some clandestine dust

of unknown provenance

a swarm of startled birds

a hundred buttons to be buttoned

crutches, walking sticks, and canes

in irregular form

*

The tender, nightgowned girl

wobbles on her base

the plastic girl twirls on cue

and then some ghosts came in on papery feet

and could not be contained

*

In a forest made from paper

that bends, breaks, repairs

I lived inside a ring of brambles

constructed to enable leaps

for the next dancer

*

This confession written by myself

using preexisting phrases

recounts the history of dirt

which was inadmissible

ACCRUAL

Italicized words borrowed from Cathy Caruth's writings

She felt a loosening. Like
being touched. Or falling down

inside the dark. Almost a dark
joy. Almost a hymn to joy. As if one could
claim one's own

survival and stop protecting
the little fragment that already has

a protective shield. The chip. The stain.
Her arms and shoulders felt tired.

And then the stuck knob that
never could be grasped
                            fell off

and she went out to watch
waves against the rocks, the plumes
diffusing into air.

And then she was in a room,
the bulky, out-of-date furniture
still there but invisible
in the dark.

To have survived means
having been compelled to make *endless*
testimony to impossibility.
Let her *wake from the dream*

and *out of death* into
having *survived, precisely, without knowing it*

so she can learn again
                    what it is

not to have survived, the dumb luck
of having been *one moment too late.*

KEATSIAN

Again the world imposes itself, impure
and redolent, filled with dimming
light, those greedy bees
                              aware

and unaware of winter's imminence.
As if to die

were just to walk into the water
fully clothed, the fabric
endlessly absorbing that element because
that is its purpose. Why not stand

a little longer in the shallows, touching
the abyss for practice, the clammy,
almost bodily feel of whatever's

in the dark container.
                              The dying
patriarch in movies rasps his gratitude
and love, his ruined voice a signal

the body is ready to be sloughed off.
But in real life, the body's requirements

come first and last. Suffering's
what's left over,
                              little
backwards math problem in which

subtraction comes first, unconveyable
handswirl
              in the air.

ACKNOWLEDGMENTS

Grateful acknowledgment is made to the publishers of the following journals, in which some of these poems originally appeared, at times in different form or with different titles:

Beloit Poetry Journal: "Ash"

Crazyhorse: "Amends," "Residue," "Unloveable"

Dogwood: "Echo," "Estrangement"

Gettysburg Review: "Displaced," "Ultimatum"

Missouri Review Online: "Envoy," "Profusion"

Red Rock Review: "Nest," "Opaque"

Rogue Agent: "Sycamore"

Southwest Review: "Concordance"

Tampa Review: "Inscribed"

Third Coast: "Announcement"

Water-Stone: "Transmutation"

Yale Review: "Unconscious"

Earlier versions of "Envoy," "Nest," and "Opaque" were included in *November Wasps*, a limited edition chapbook published by Finishing Line Press.

Thanks to the Nevada Council for the Arts, the University of Nevada, Reno, College of Liberal Arts Scholarly and Creative Activities Grant Program and UNR's English Department for funding to support the writing of this book, and to the CAMAC, Centrum, Ucross, and Wellspring Foundations for residencies during which some of this collection's poems were written and revised.

Thanks too to the Center for the History of Medicine at Harvard's Countway Library and to Guillaume Delaunay of the Bibliothèque Universitaire Pitié / Bibliothèque Charcot in Paris for research assistance with the history of hysteria. And thanks to readers of this manuscript, especially Julia Lisella, Martha Serpas, Lisa Sewell, and the staff and participants at the Colrain Manuscript Workshop.

About the Author

Ann Keniston is the author of two earlier poetry collections, *The Caution of Human Gestures* (David Robert Books, 2005), and a chapbook, *November Wasps: Elegies* (Finishing Line, 2013). She is also the coeditor of *The New American Poetry of Engagement: A 21st Century Anthology* (McFarland, 2012). A recipient of fellowships and grants in poetry from the Nevada Arts Council, Sierra Arts (Reno), and the Somerville (MA) Arts Council, she has held residencies at the CAMAC Arts Center (France), the Ucross Foundation, the Ragdale Foundation, the Blue Mountain Center, and elsewhere. Her poems have appeared in numerous journals, including the *Yale Review, Gettysburg Review, Water-Stone*, and *Literary Imagination*. A frequent teacher of poetry in K-12 classes, she has also taught poetry and publishing workshops in the community. She is a professor of English at the University of Nevada, Reno, where she teaches poetry workshops and literature classes.

www.annkeniston.com